To My Uncle Yves ~ My heart is overwhelmed by your memory. I will live with your love and guidance forever.

In Honor of Gary and Emmanuel Daphnis.

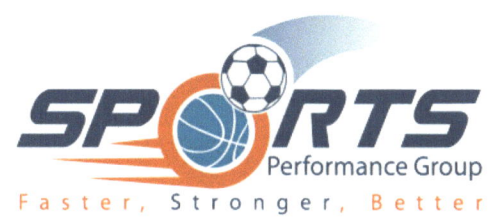

Editing and Design by Karen Riccio

For further information and products, please visit us at Theathletesbodywithin.com.

Follow us on Facebook and Twitter.

Disclaimer

You must get your physician's approval before beginning this exercise/nutrition program.

The recommendations in this book are not medical guidelines but are for educational purposes only. You must consult your physician prior to starting this program or if you have any medical condition or injury that contraindicates physical activity or if you are taking any medications. This program is designed for healthy individuals 18 years and older only.

The dietary programs in this book are not intended as a substitute for any exercise routine or treatment or dietary regimen that may have been prescribed by your physician.

You must have a complete physical examination if you are sedentary or overweight, have high cholesterol, high blood pressure, or diabetes, or if you are over 30 years old. Please discuss all nutritional changes with your physician or a registered dietician.

Before beginning any diet and exercise program, please consult your physician. The author disclaims any liability, express or implied, resulting from the application or misapplication of any of the information in any *The Athlete's Body Within* guide.

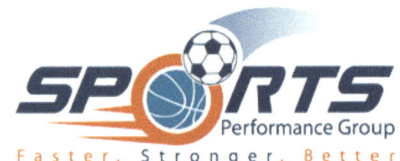

Have fun getting to know the new you!

The New You

The Athlete's Body Within is dedicated to restoring, maintaining and optimizing, as quickly and effectively as possible, the physical and mental capacities of those, like us, who want to look like the athlete we imagine within ourselves . Our goal is to decrease and/or avoid needless aches and pains and increase each person's ability to become more mobile, strong and athletic. We will focus on all the means to recover and find the athletic body within and seek to provide this information to the public at large.

Contents:

- The New You...... pages 4-5
- How SMART Are You...... pages 6-8
- Setting Goals...... Pages 9-14
- What Stands in Your Way...... pages 15-16
- Managing Stress...... Pages 17-18
- Having Fun...... Page 19

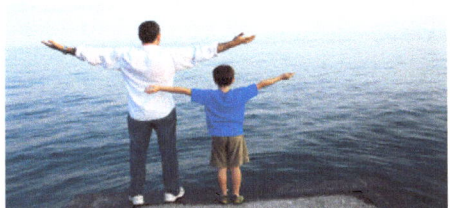

"What lies behind us and what lies before us are tiny matters compared to what lies within us."
Ralph Waldo Emerson

The New You

Here you are! At the start of a new you! Sometimes the start is easy. It's staying on track, staying motivated, that's so tough. In this manual you will learn how to stay motivated and on your path. But remember, only **you** have the power to use the information you learn.

It is impossible to know absolutely everything about fitness; no one does. But, we do know how to lose weight and the information contained in this manual will teach you just that. Before you start this program remember these two things:

1. **You will learn more about yourself through this whole process than you ever imagined.** Weight loss is purely a system; the rest is a test of mental and physical strength. You will learn about your strengths and weaknesses through this process.

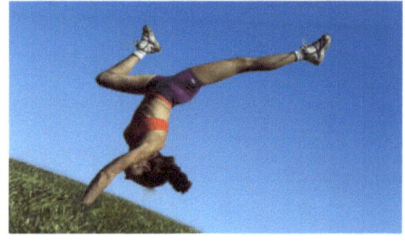

"Though no one can go back and make a brand new start, anyone can start from now and make a brand new ending."
Carl Bard

The New You

2. **You control your own destiny.** Do not feed into the scientific ranting about genetics. Genetics are decisive factors for hair color, skin color, and things that we cannot control. You can control what your body looks like.

So let's get started. Make sure to read this entire manual so you don't miss a thing. If you encounter any problems, have any questions, or just want to tell someone about your success, make sure to e-mail us at: info@theathletesbodywithin.com. You can also become a fan on Facebook. Visit us at www.theathletesbodywithin.com and tell us your success stories and upload your amazing before and after photos.

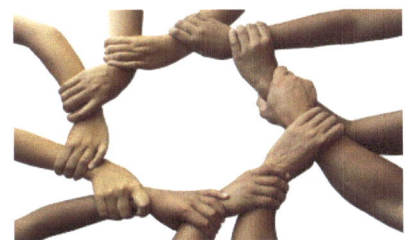

> *"Motivation is a fire from within. If someone else tries to light that fire under you, chances are it will burn very briefly."*
> **Stephen R. Covey**

How SMART Are You?

Staying with your Exercise Program

It feels good to be in control of your exercise habits. Perhaps you've started a program and are making strides towards a life-time of regular exercise. What steps or strategies can you use to make sure you stay with your exercise program?

We use the SMART Strategy:

Specific. Narrow down what you hope to achieve. When and how will you accomplish your goal? Determine small milestones along the way and celebrate when you reach them. How about a race? Gather your co-workers and sign up for some classes or a fun run. Feel great about yourself by doing well at the company 5k or finishing your first marathon.

Measurable. How can you determine improvement? Include ways to gauge your success. This could be amount of time spent exercising, measurement of your body fat, distance traveled when exercising, pounds lifted, classes attended, etc.

Achievable. Make sure your goals are realistic – before you can run a marathon you should start with something shorter. Your local running club has plenty of events for you to chose from (55 meters to the marathon). Set a goal that is reachable, yet causes you to go beyond what you're currently doing.

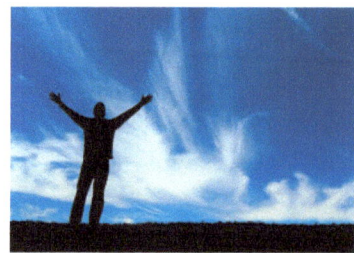

"I'm not telling you it is going to be easy - I'm telling you it's going to be worth it"
Art Williams

How SMART Are You?

SMART Strategy continued

Relevant. The goal has to be important to **you**. Examine your inner motivation and be passionate about what you want to achieve.

Timely. Success doesn't happen overnight – it takes time and effort. Break your goal into manageable segments with a realistic time frame for accomplishing each.

Staying Focused

It's easy to get bored doing the same thing every day. Freshen up your exercise routine to avoid getting in a rut. Think of ways to add some excitement to your workout:

- **Try a new activity or sport.**
- **Vary your intensity level.**
- **Join a group playing a sport in your town.**
- **Change the order and length of your exercises.**

"Most people are average because they do average things..."

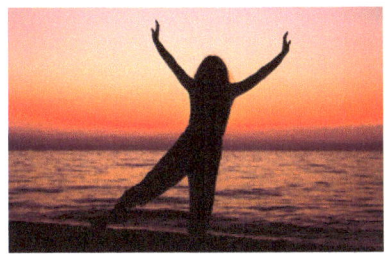

"When you get to the end of your rope, tie a knot and hang on."
Franklin D. Roosevelt

How SMART Are You?

IMPORTANT INFO:

Did you know...

The average cost of a gym membership is $54.00 a month. This may seem expensive, but did you know...

Regular exercise would save the average person $72.00 a month in medical bills caused by not being physically fit. By exercising, you can save $18.00 a month. You can see that in less than a year you will save over $210.00 from the benefits of a healthier body.

Work Ethic:

There are many workout programs that can and will help you. The program we have set up is what we have seen work in the past through our own experiences as well as what we have seen through the experiences of others.

We will provide the information and resources you need to accomplish your goals, but only you can motivate yourself to acheive them. There are many steps to take to create your ideal body. If you follow the steps we have provided, we can guarantee success. But that's all up to you.

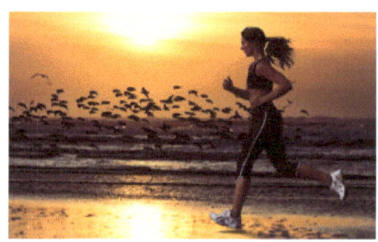

"People often say that motivation doesn't last. Well, neither does bathing - that's why we recommend it daily."
Zig Ziglar

Setting Goals

If you want to lose weight, you must figure out how you are going to get there. Figuring out the path to weight loss is called your direction. This book will give you that direction. But you need a place to go, somewhere to end. You eventually want to reach a final point. This is called your goal; it is what you have set out to achieve. Here is a little bit about goals...

Long-term goals:

Long-term goals are those aspirations that you have to work for, ones that you know will take some work but that you would like to accomplish. Here are examples of three goals for someone who is trying to lose weight:

1. **Lose 10 pounds in 6 weeks.**
2. **Reduce my body fat by 3%.**
3. **Eat right so I get the best results.**

These are your *long-term goals* and should be aimed at something that you know you can reach over a period of time. Do not make goals that are unreachable because you will feel overwhelmed as you realize they are unattainable.

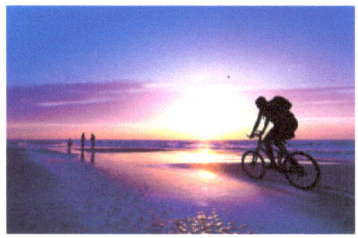

"It's lack of faith that makes people afraid of meeting challenges, and I believed in myself."
Muhammed Ali

Setting Goals

Short-term goals:

Short-term goals are the week-to-week aspirations that you need to accomplish to reach your long-term goals. Here would be an example of some short-term fitness goals:

1. **Workout everyday before I go to work from 7:00AM-8:15AM.**
2. **Pack my meals so I know that I am eating right.**
3. **Track my daily & weekly progress.**
4. **Eat 6 meals everyday.**

Daily and weekly goals are called *short-term goals* and are necessary to reach your *long-term goals*. Using this system will bring you closer to the body you desire.

Remember, without goals you have no guidance or focus on where you are going, and it is very easy to lose sight of what you set out to do.

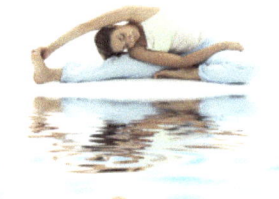

" Accomplishing a goal is not as important as the person you become accomplishing it."
Neil Armstrong

Setting Goals

Take a few minutes now and think about why you purchased this manual. Think back to the website, everything you read and what it was that finally talked you into purchasing this system. Try to remember, reading the information on the website. If you can't remember go back to the website and read it again.

There was a reason you bought this system, and whatever that reason was could probably be turned into a goal. If this book was a gift, there was a reason it was given to you. Maybe you're interested in the subject or you would like to lose some weight. Whatever your reason was, you are here right now.

Now take out a pen and write down three long-term goals and three short-term goals related to fitness that you would like to see happen for you. What do you want to do with your body? *Lose weight? Tone up? Get Stronger?* Take your time when you make your lists. Really focus on what you want.

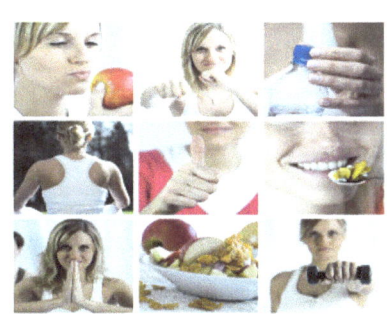

"*I am not discouraged, because every wrong attempt discarded is another step forward.*"
Thomas A. Edison

Setting Goals

My Long-Term Fitness Goals:

1.

2.

3.

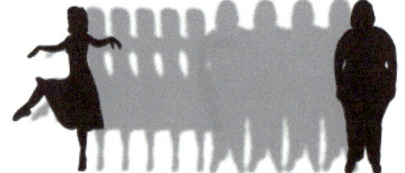

"Opportunity is missed by most
people because it is dressed in
overalls and looks like work."
Thomas A. Edison

Setting Goals

My Short-Term Fitness Goals:

1.

2.

3.

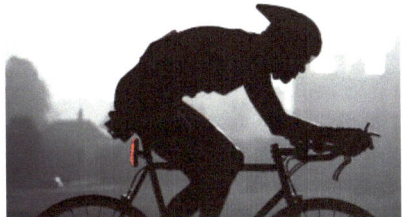

"The only time you mustn't fail is the last time you try."
Charles F. Kettering

Setting Goals

Now, take these two lists and hang them in your bathroom. You will see them every day right when you get up in the morning and right before you go to bed.

You will be reminded of your fitness goals all day and all night. Your subconscious will take these thoughts and it will process them until they become real. This is very important if you want to accomplish this test of mental and physical strength.

Announce Your Goals:

This might be the hardest part! Accountability! If you really want this program to work, you must make a public commitment by telling three people your goals. Think of three people that you see once a day or a few times a week. These people will be very helpful to you. On the following lines, write down the names and phone numbers of the three people you are going to call:

Name_____ Phone #_____

Name_____ Phone #_____

Name_____ Phone #_____

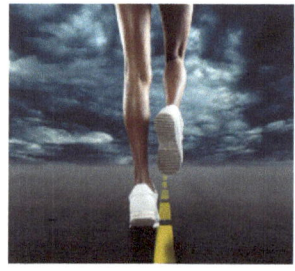

"People with goals succeed because they know where they are going. It's as simple as that."
Earl Nightingale

What Stands In Your Way?

Recognize possible obstacles:

With everything that we do in life, something always seems to come up. These "things" that come up interfere with who we want to be and where we want to go in life. Some people love to sleep in. That creates certain obstacles right at the start of your day! You have to recognize the obstacle and then change the behavior. Not so easy, huh?

Currently, there are some obstacles in your fitness path; otherwise you would already have the body you desire. In order to achieve our goals we need to recognize our obstacles. And isn't it ironic that we tend to get in our own ways most of the time? Well, there's no sense in doing that at all. This is the time to stay focused and keep all obstacles to a minimum.

Take a few minutes and think about what is getting in your way as it relates to exercise. Is it an eating habit, a sleeping habit, or maybe exercising just wasn't important to you in the past? Think about what is standing in your way.

On the next page, write down three possible obstacles that may have prevented you from achieving your goals in the past.

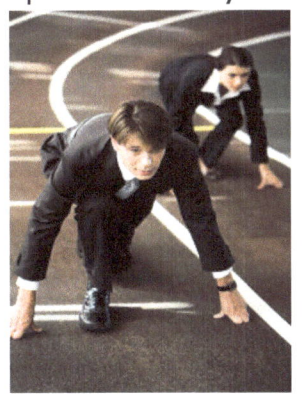

"Nothing will ever be attempted if all possible objections must first be overcome."
Samuel Johnson

What Stands In Your Way?

3 Possible Obstacles:

1. _____

_____

2. _____

_____

3. _____

_____

Now that you have recognized these obstacles, make a commitment to change these three behaviors so you can achieve your goals. If you have a bad eating habit, make an extra effort to fix it. If you can overcome obstacles, it will be smooth sailing until you have a great looking physique.

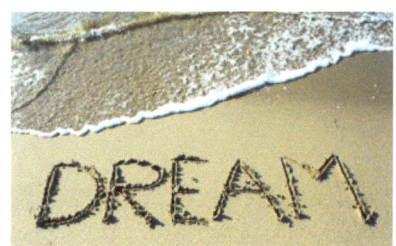

"Patience and perseverance have a magical effect before which difficulties disappear and obstacles vanish."
John Quincy Adam

Managing Stress

Managing Stress:

Stress is your body responding to change. This can be a positive response or negative, depending on the situation. A situation that one person finds stressful may not bother someone else. For example, one person may become anxious when traveling, while another person may find traveling a source of relaxation. Things that cause fear in some people, such as adventure sports, may be fun for others. Each of us reacts differently to the stress we encounter.

Stress can be a positive influence in our lives when managed properly. Speaking to a group of people, watching a great sporting event, or cycling down a challenging trail can be stressful, but also fun! Life would be very dull without some stress. The key is to manage stress properly, because too much of it can lead to health problems in some people.

Stress Can:

 -make you feel angry, afraid, agitated or helpless.
 -keep you awake at night.
 -give you aches and pains throughout your body.
 -lead to habits such as smoking, drinking, overeating, and drug abuse.

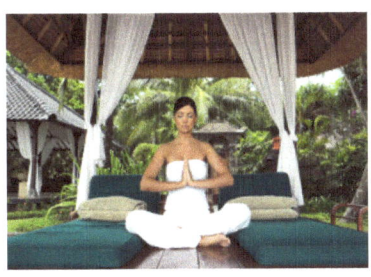

"People become really quite remarkable when they start thinking that they can do things. When they believe in themselves they have the first secret of success."
Norman Vincent Peale

Managing Stress

Outside influences affect us every minute of every day. It is not the outside forces but how you react inside that's important. You can't control all of the outside events in your life, but you can change how you handle them emotionally and psychologically.

Strategies for Managing Stress:

- Try to accept things you can't change. Talk out your troubles and look for the good in situations.
- Exercise regularly. Walk, swim, ride a bike, run or use an elliptical machine to get a sustained workout using big muscle groups. Exercise helps you let go of stress and tension, leaving you feeling a lot better.
- Learn to say no to others and to **yourself**. Don't promise too much. Give yourself time to get things done.
- Try to take 5 to 10 minutes each day to breathe deeply. You have to not only focus on taking deep breaths but also letting out long, deep breaths.
- Limit nicotine, sodas and alcohol.

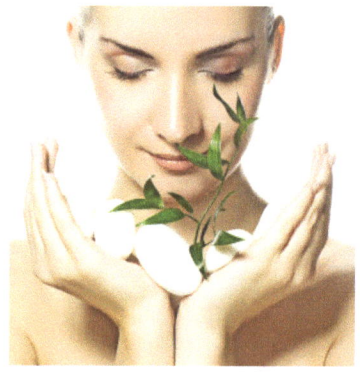

"You have a very powerful mind that can make anything happen as long as you keep yourself centered."
Dr. Wayne W. Dyer

Having Fun

Having Fun:

It seems like every time you pick up a book that has anything to do with fitness, it never says a word about having fun. The people in the pictures demonstrating the exercises have absolutely no trace of a smile on their faces.

There are 2 kinds of fun:

  1. Having fun building your house.
  2. Having fun at a theme park.

Getting your body into shape is like "building your house" type of fun. There is a lot of hard work that is involved. But when you get the final result you are extremely happy about what you have accomplished and it is very enjoyable. The feeling of accomplishment stays with you as you enjoy your house everyday!

So, be happy and have fun when you workout. Have a friend come with you to the gym, or make friends at the gym. Laugh and smile as you are working hard to get the body you desire; it will make time pass very quickly. Whatever you have to do to have fun, do it. Be creative, never get embarrassed, and it will make time fly!

You're on your way now! Revisit sections of this manual whenever you need to refocus and stay strong!

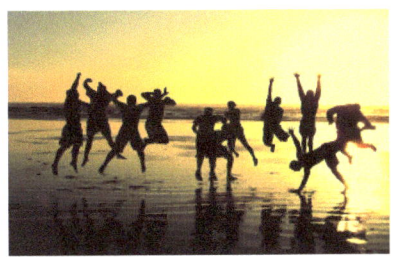

"Only those who risk going too far can possibly find out how far one can go."
T.S. Eliot

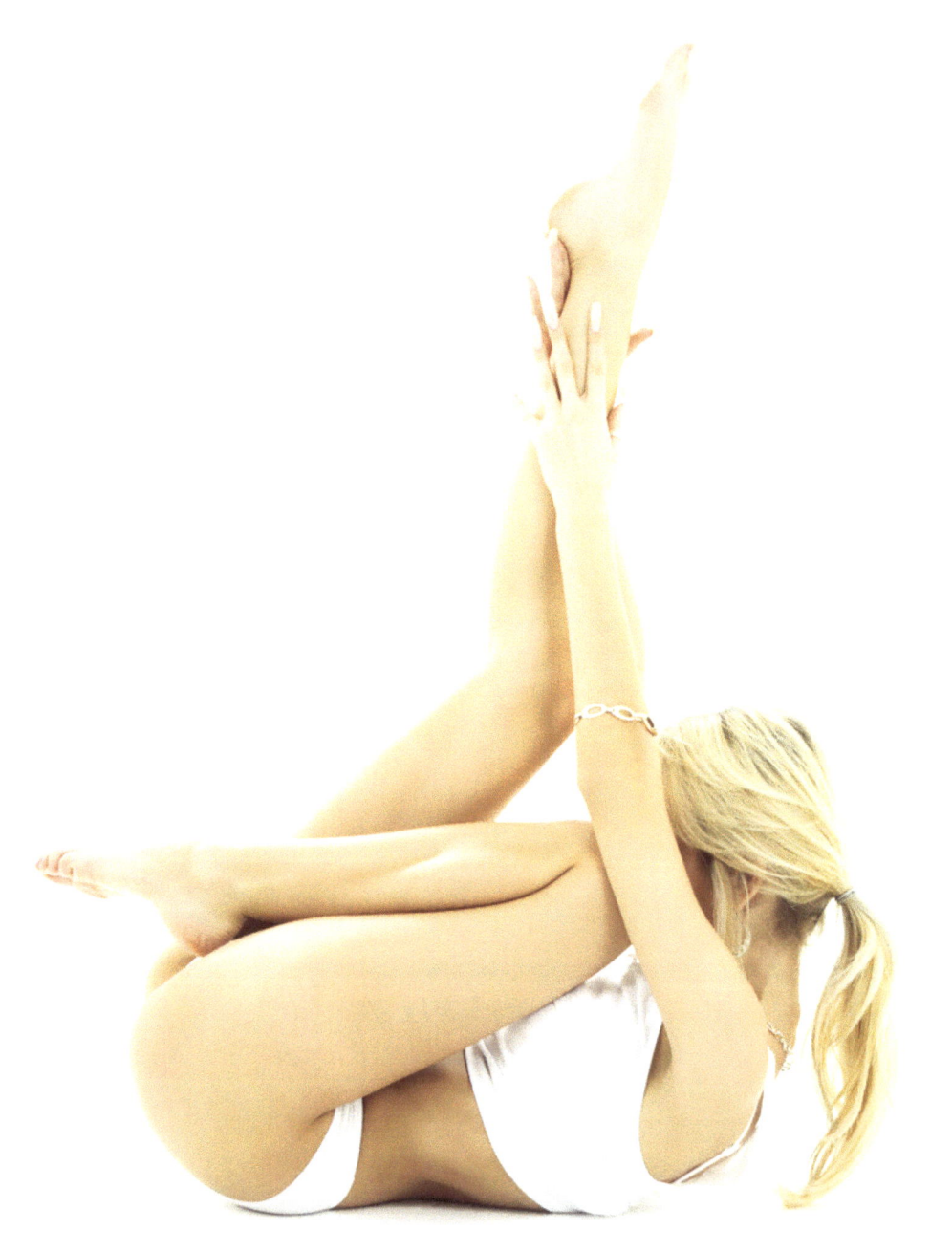

The conscious brain can only hold one thought at a time. Choose a positive thought.

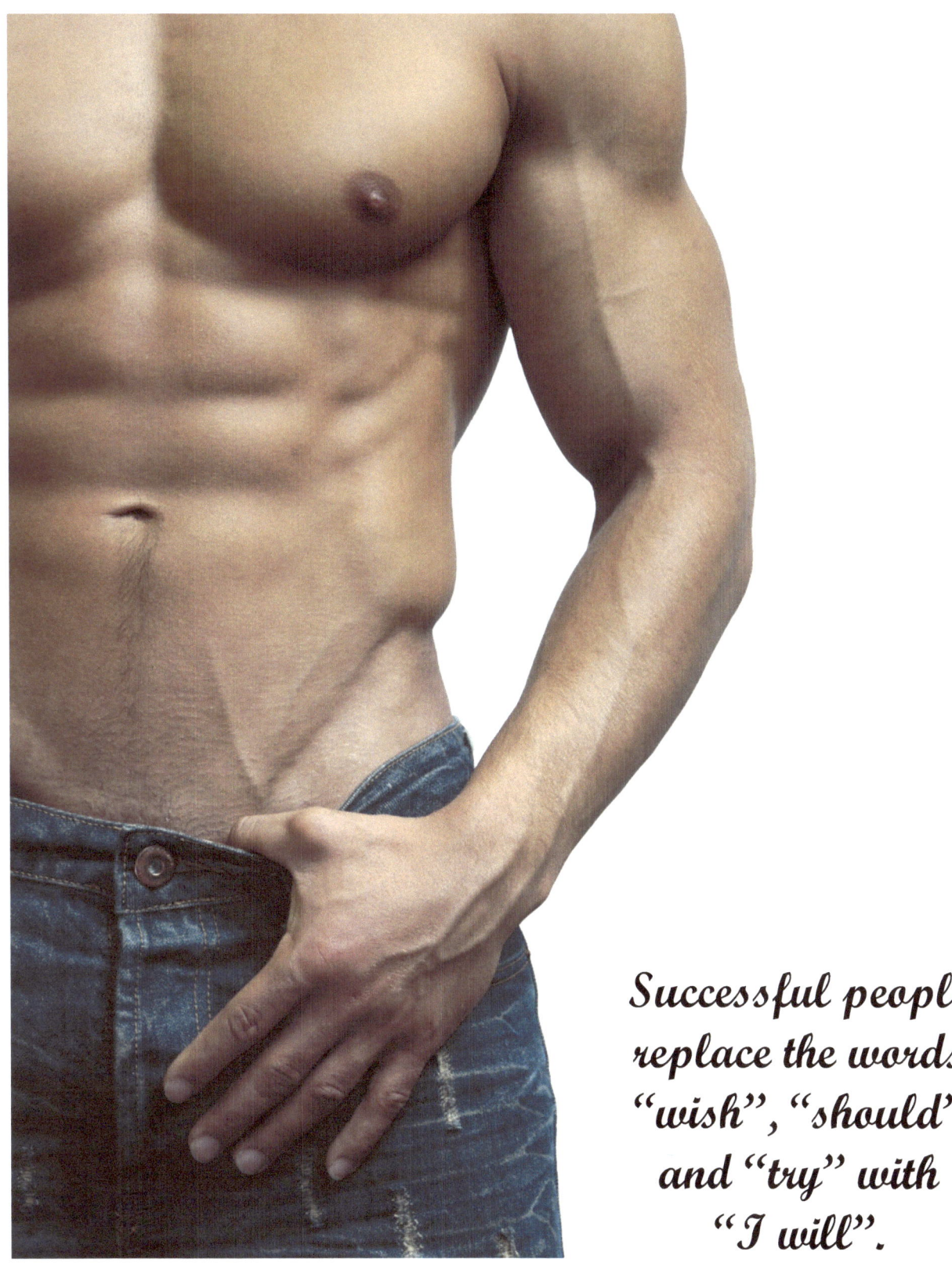

Successful people replace the words "wish", "should" and "try" with "I will".

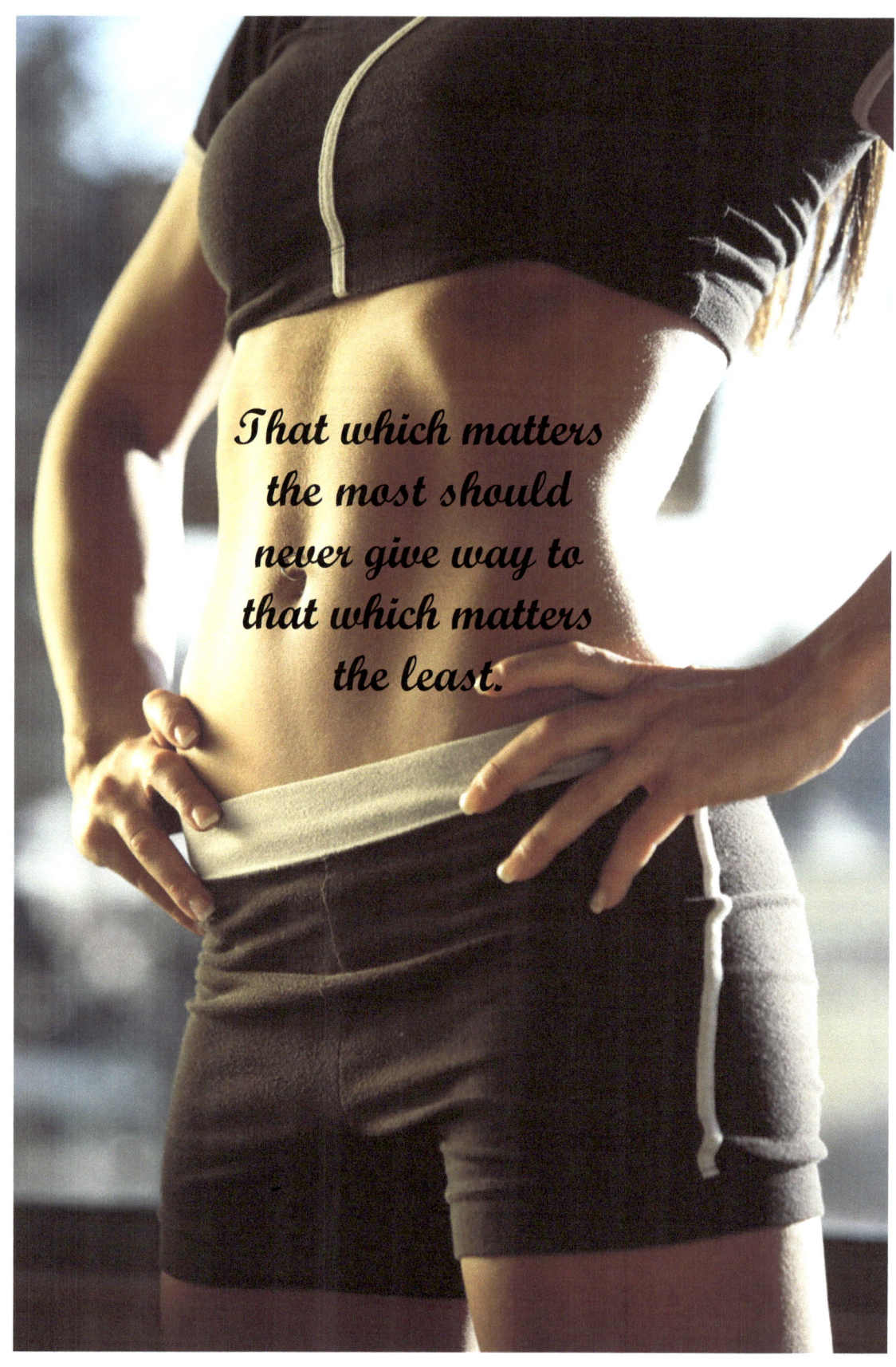

That which matters
the most should
never give way to
that which matters
the least.

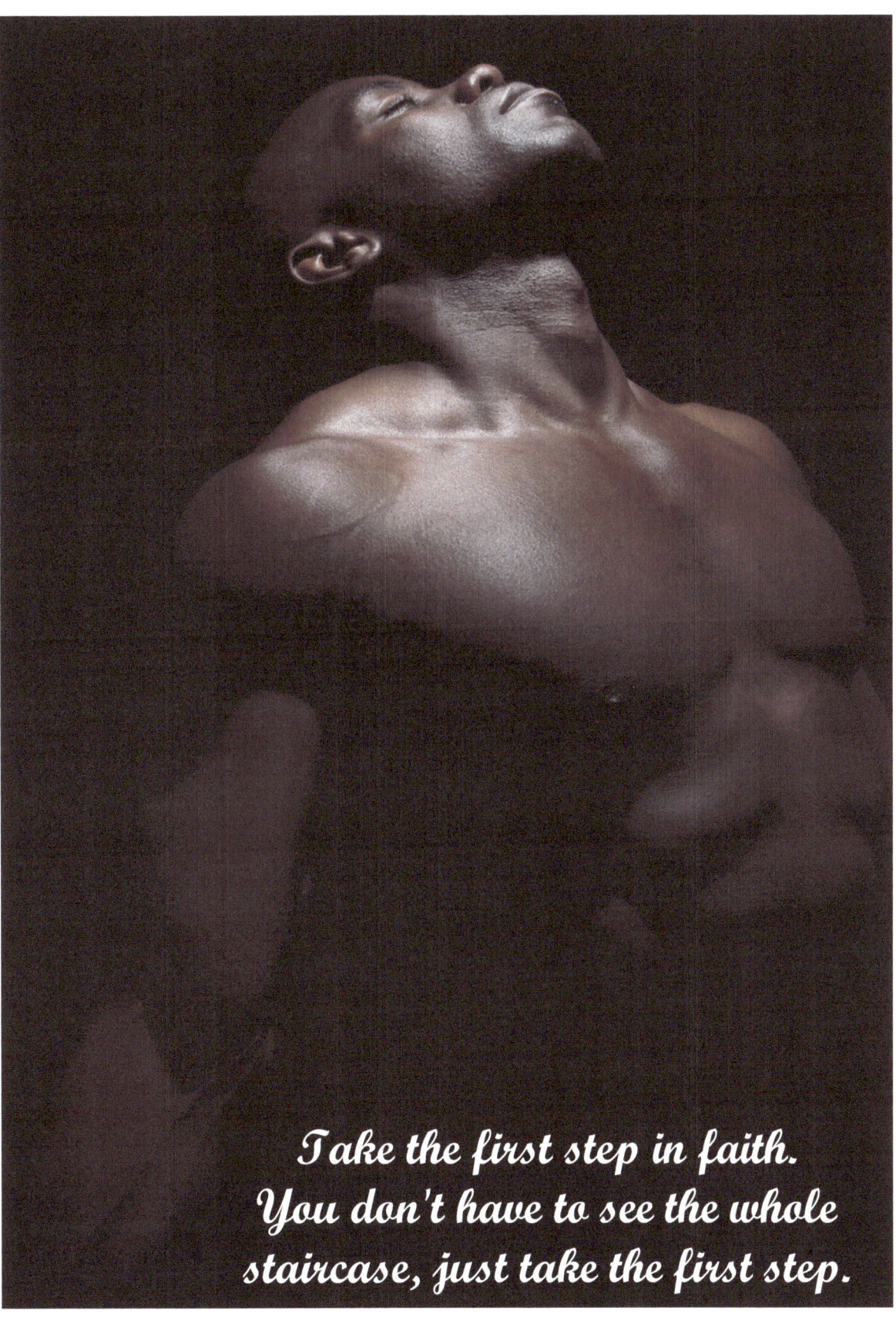

Take the first step in faith.
You don't have to see the whole
staircase, just take the first step.

Congratulations!
You have the motivation now!
Your next step is to uncover your inner athlete with
The Preparation Phase and
The Nutrition Handbook.
Order your copies today at www.theathletesbodywithin.com
The Athlete's Body Within

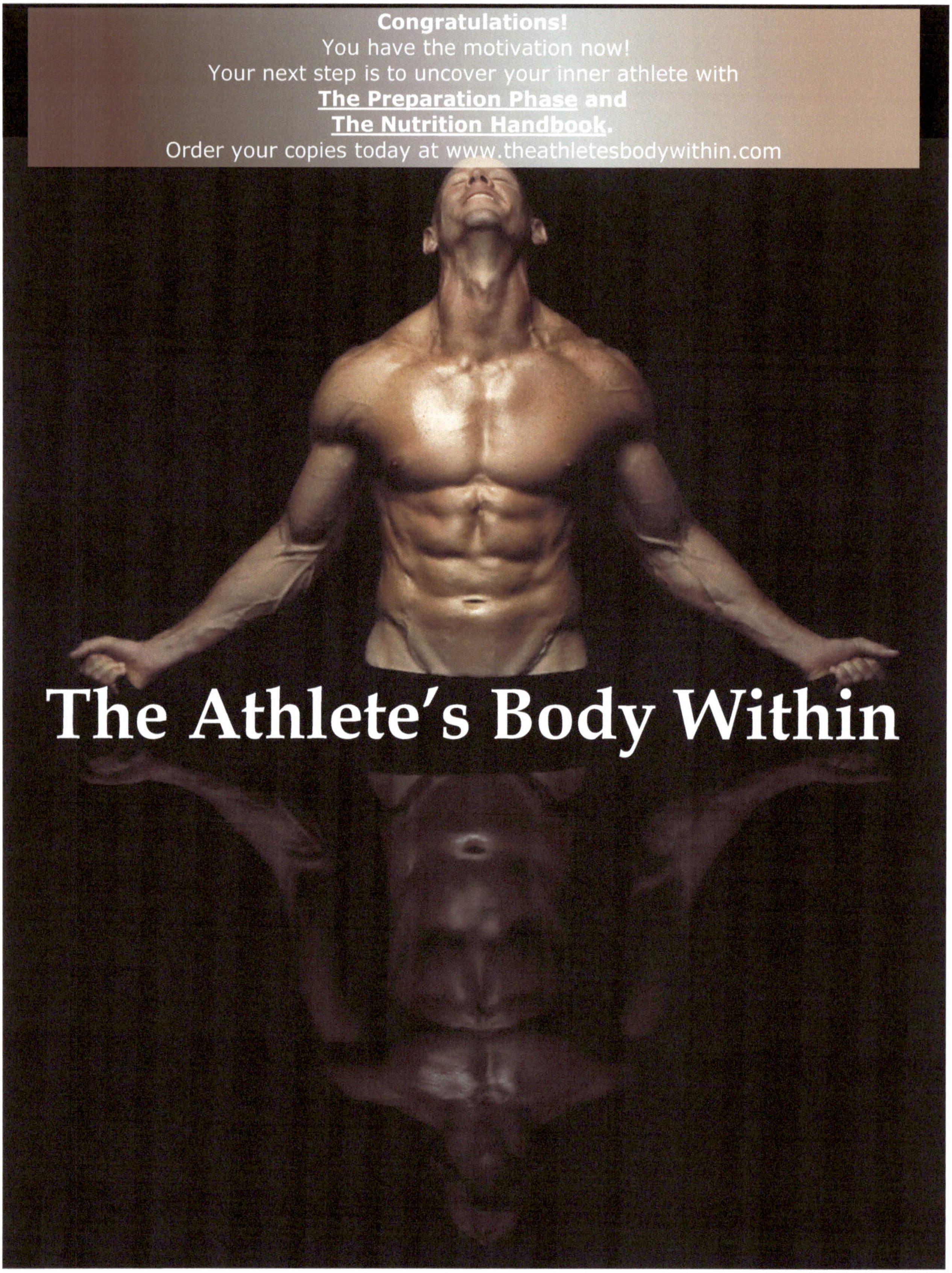

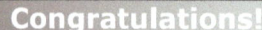

www.ingramcontent.com/pod-product-compliance
Lightning Source LLC
Chambersburg PA
CBHW060825290526
45792CB00005BB/1804